Air Fryer Cookbook for Beginners

50 Amazing and Simple Recipes to Prepare in Your Air Fryer
By
Elena Brown

This document is geared towards
providing exact and reliable
information in regards to the topic
and issue covered. The publication is
sold with the idea that the publisher
is not required to render accounting,
officially permitted or otherwise
qualified services. If advice is
necessary, legal or professional, a
practiced individual in the
profession should be ordered.

From a Declaration of Principles
which was accepted and approved
equally by a Committee of the
American Bar Association and a
Committee of Publishers and
Associations.

The information provided herein is
stated to be truthful and consistent,
in that any liability, in terms of
inattention or otherwise, by any
usage or abuse of any policies,

Table of Contents

Introduction

Air fryers are full of hot air, and that's the best thing about them. They are basically small, powerful ovens, and ovens use air as the vehicle for heat, while frying uses fat as the vehicle for heat.

Because air fryers are ovens and not fryers, the food that comes out of your fryer will not be 100% identical to the onion rings at Cone-n-Shake or the calamari rings at your favorite bar and grill.

The result is that air fryers are much less messy and require much less oil than run-of-the-mill fryers.

Even better, these little ovens can do much more than producing fake fried food. Air fryers bring beautifully browned vegetables, crackly-skinned chicken wings, and even light, airy pies all to your fingertips.

The Different Types of Air Fryers

The most common type of air fryer on the market, the basket-type air fryer, looks like a funky coffee pot with a removable basket in its belly. This air fryer has only one function: air frying. This guide covers basket-type air fryers.

You can also find boxed multifunction air fryers on the market. They look like toaster ovens on steroids, and air frying is just one of the things they do (between slow cooking, dehydrating, and toasting). They also have more food holding capacity than basket-type air fryers.

Important Tips to Keep in Mind when Using an Air Fryer

- **Always have the rack in the basket.** This allows hot air to circulate around the food and also prevents the food from sitting in excess oil.

- **Air fryers are noisy.** When it is running, you will hear buzzing from the fans.
- **Handy.** Even browning requires you to remove the basket and mix the food every few minutes.
- **It's okay to take the basket out to take a look.** You can do this at any time during the cooking process. It is not necessary to turn the machine off, as it shuts itself off when the basket is out.
- **Consequently, make sure the drawer is fully inserted or it will not turn back on.** You'll know, because the air fryer will suddenly be silent.
- **Food cooks fast, faster than you're used to!** This is one of the best attributes of the air fryer. Your air fryer manual probably has a helpful chart of cooking times and temperatures for common foods. The less food in the

basket, the shorter the cooking time; the more food, the longer it will be.

- **You may need a slightly lower temperature.** Many air fryer recipes call for lower temperature settings than their conventional counterparts. This may seem suspicious, but go with it. Again, air fryers heat up very fast and move that hot air, so a slightly lower temperature will help prevent food from building up. also dark or crispy on the outside, while cooking properly on the inside.

Chapter 1. Breakfast Recipes

1. Egg Muffins

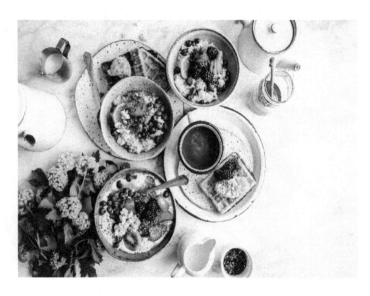

(Ready in about 25 mins | Serving 1 | Easy)

Ingredients:

- 1 egg

- 2 tablespoons of olive oil

- 3 tablespoons of milk

- 3.5 ounces of white flour

- 1 tablespoon of baking powder

- 2 ounces of parmesan, grated

- A splash of Worcestershire sauce

Directions:

1. Mix the egg and starch, butter, baking powder, cheese, and parmesan in a pot, stir well, and split into 4 cups of silicon muffin.
2. Arrange cups, cover, and cook at 392° F for 15 minutes in the cooking basket of your AirFryer.
3. For breakfast, serve warm.
4. Enjoy!

Nutrition: Calories: 251, Fat: 6g, Fiber: 8g, Carbs: 9g, Protein: 3g.

2. Polenta Bites

(Ready in about 30 mins | Serving 4 | Normal)

Ingredients:

For the polenta:

- 1 tablespoon of butter

- 1 cup of cornmeal

- 3 cups of water

- Salt and black pepper to the taste

For the polenta bites:

- 2 tablespoons of powdered sugar

- Cooking spray

Directions:

1. Mix water in a saucepan with cornmeal, sugar, salt, and pepper, stir, bring to a boil over medium heat, simmer

for 10 minutes, take off heat, whisk again and hold in the refrigerator until it is cool.

2. Scoop 1 spoonful of polenta, shape a ball and place it on a working surface.
3. Repeat with the rest of the polenta, place all the balls in your AirFryer's cooking tub, sprinkle them with cooking oil, cover, and steam for 8 minutes at 380° F.
4. Arrange bits of polenta on bowls, scatter sugar all over, and serve as toast.
5. Enjoy!

Nutrition: Calories: 231, Fat: 7g, Fiber: 8g, Carbs: 12g, Protein: 4g.

3. Delicious Breakfast Potatoes

(Ready in about 30 mins | Serving 4 | Normal)

Ingredients:

- 2 tablespoons of olive oil

- 3 potatoes, cubed

- 1 yellow onion, chopped

- 1 red bell pepper, chopped

- Salt and black pepper to the taste

- 1 teaspoon of garlic powder

- 1 teaspoon of sweet paprika

- 1 teaspoon of onion powder

Directions:

1. Grease the basket of your AirFryer with olive oil, add

the potatoes, mix with salt and pepper, and season.

2. Remove onion, bell pepper, garlic powder, paprika, and onion powder, then mix properly, cover, and simmer for 30 minutes at 370° F.

3. Place potatoes on plates and serve as a snack.

Nutrition: Calories: 214, Fat: 6g, Fiber: 8g, Carbs: 15g, Protein: 4g.

4. Tasty Cinnamon Toast

(Preparation time: 10 min | Cooking time: 5 min | Servings: 6)

Ingredients:

- 1 stick of butter, soft
- 12 bread slices
- ½ cup of sugar
- 1 and ½ teaspoon of vanilla extract
- 1 and ½ teaspoon of cinnamon powder

Directions:

1. Mix the soft butter and the honey, and cinnamon in a cup and whisk well.
2. Spread this on slices of bread, put them in your fryer, and cook for 5 minutes at 400° F
3. Serve for breakfast and split between dishes.

4. Enjoy!
Nutrition: Calories: 221, Fat: 4g,
Fiber: 7g, Carbs: 12g, Protein: 8g.

5. Delicious Potato Hash

(Ready in about 30 mins | Serving 4 | Normal)

Ingredients:

- 1 and ½ potatoes, cubed

- 1 yellow onion, chopped

- 2 teaspoons of olive oil

- 1 green bell pepper, chopped

- Salt and black pepper to the taste

- ½ teaspoon of dried thyme

- 2 eggs

Directions:

1. Heat the AirFryer to 350° F, add butter, heat it, add onion, bell pepper, salt, and pepper, stir and cook for 5 minutes.

2. Add the onions, thyme, and peas. Stir, cover, and simmer for 20 minutes at 360° F.
3. Serve for breakfast.
4. Enjoy!

Nutrition: Calories: 241, Fat: 4g, Fiber: 7g, Carbs: 12g, Protein: 7g.

Chapter 2. Sides, Snacks and Appetizers Recipes

6. Mini Sweet Pepper

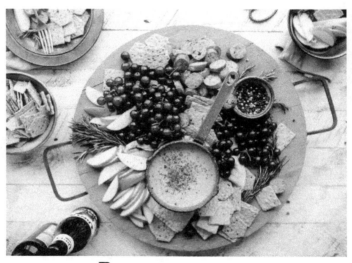

Poppers

(Ready in about 30 min | Servings 4 | Yields 16 halves (4 per serving) | Normal)

Ingredients:

- 8 mini sweet peppers

- 4 ounces of full-Fat: cream cheese, softened

- 4 slices of sugar-free bacon, cooked and crumbled

- 1/4 cup of shredded pepper jack cheese

Directions:

1. Cut the pepper tops and slice on half lengthwise each. To cut seeds and membranes using a small knife.
2. Put together the cream cheese, bacon, and pepper jack in a shallow tub.
3. In each sweet pepper, put 3 teaspoons of the mixture and press smoothly hard — place in basket fryer.
4. Set the temperature to 400° F, and set the timer for eight minutes.
5. Serve sweet and enjoy!

Nutrition: Calories: 176, Protein: 7.4g, Fiber: 0.9g Net Carbohydrates: 2.7g Fat: 13.4g, Sodium: 309 mg, Carbohydrates: 3.6 g sugar: 2.2g.

7. Spicy Spinach Artichoke Dip

(Ready in about 20 min | Servings 6 | Easy)

Ingredients:

- 10 ounces of frozen spinach, drained and thawed

- 1 (14-ounce) can of artichoke hearts, drained and chopped

- 1/4 cup of chopped pickled jalapeños

- 8 ounces of full-Fat: cream cheese, softened

- 1/4 cup of full-Fat: mayonnaise

- 1/4 cup of full-Fat: sour cream

- 1/2 teaspoon of garlic powder

- ¼ cup of grated Parmesan cheese

- 1 cup of shredded pepper jack cheese

Directions:

1. Combine the ingredients in a 4-cup baking dish. Put the basket into the AirFryer.
2. Set the temperature to 320° F and change the timer for 10 minutes.
3. Start as orange, then bubble. Serve fresh and enjoy!

Nutrition: Calories: 226, Protein: 10.0g, Fiber: 3.7g, Net Carbohydrates: 6.5g Fat: 15.9g, Sodium: 776 mg, Carbohydrates: 10.2g sugar: 3.4g.

8. Personal Mozzarella Pizza Crust

(Ready in about 15 min | Servings 1 | Normal)

Ingredients:

- 1/2 cup of shredded whole-milk mozzarella cheese

- 2 tablespoons of blanched finely ground almond flour

- 1 tablespoon of full-Fat: cream cheese

- 1 large egg white

Directions:

1. In a medium microwave-safe bowl, place the mozzarella, almond flour, and cream cheese. Microwave that lasted 30 seconds. Stir until the dough ball forms smoothly. Add egg white and stir until the dough forms soft and round.

2. Press the crust of a 6 round pizza.
3. Cut a piece of parchment to fit your AirFryer basket and place the crust on the parchment.
4. Set the temperature to 350° F and adjust the timer for 10 minutes.
5. Flip over the crust after 5 minutes and place any desired toppings at this time. Continue to cook until golden. Serve immediately.

Nutrition: Calories: 314, Protein: 19.9g Fiber: 1.5g, Net Carbohydrates: 3.6g Fat: 22.7g, Sodium: 457 mg Carbohydrates: 5.1g, Sugar: 1.8g.

9. Garlic Cheese Bread

(Ready in about 20 min | Servings 2 | Easy)

Ingredients:

- 1 cup of shredded mozzarella cheese

- 1/4 cup of grated Parmesan cheese

- 1 large egg

- 1/2 teaspoon of garlic powder

Directions:

1. Mix the ingredients in a large bowl. Cut a piece of parchment to fit your basket with AirFryer. Press the mixture on the parchment in a circle, and place it in the basket of the AirFryer.
2. Set the temperature to 350° F and change the timer for 10 minutes.

3. Serve hot and enjoy!
Nutrition: Calories: 258, Protein: 19.2g Fiber: 0.1g Net Carbohydrates: 3.6g Fat: 16.6g, Sodium: 612 mg Carbohydrates: 3.7g, Sugar: 0.7g.

10. Crustless Three-Meat Pizza

(Ready in about 10 min | Servings 1 | Easy)

Ingredients:

- 1/2 cup of shredded mozzarella cheese

- 7 slices of pepperoni

- 1/4 cup of cooked ground sausage

- 2 slices of sugar-free bacon, cooked and crumbled

- 1 tablespoon of grated Parmesan cheese

- 2 tablespoons of low-carb, sugar-free pizza sauce for dipping

Directions:

1. Cover the bottom of the cake pan with mozzarella. Put the

pepperoni, sausage, and bacon on top of the cheese and sprinkle with the Parmesan. Place the pan in the basket of the AirFryer.

2. Change the temperature to 400° F and set a 5-minute timer.

3. Cut until the cheese is crispy and bubbling. Serve warm with a pizza sauce for dipping.

4. Enjoy!

Nutrition: Calories: 466, Protein: 28.1 g Fiber: 0.5 g, Net Carbohydrates: 4.7 g Fat: 34.0 g, Sodium: 1,446 mg Carbohydrates: 5.2 g, Sugar: 1.6 g.

11. Smoky BBQ Roasted Almonds

(Ready in about 11 min | Servings 2 | Easy)

Ingredients:

- 1 cup of raw almonds
- 2 teaspoons of coconut oil
- 1 teaspoon of chili powder
- 1/4 teaspoon of cumin
- 1/4 teaspoon of smoked paprika
- 1/4 teaspoon of onion powder

Directions:

1. Dump all ingredients in a wide bowl until the almonds are uniformly filled with oil and spices—place almonds in the basket for AirFryer.

2. Set the temperature to 320° F and change the timer for 6 minutes.
3. Remove the basket from the fryer halfway through the cooking time. Enable to absolutely cool off.
4. Enjoy!

Nutrition: Calories: 182, Protein: 6.2 g, Fiber: 3.3 g, Net Carbohydrates: 3.3 g Fat: 16.3 g, Sodium: 19 mg, Carbohydrates: 6.6 g sugar: 1.1 g.

12. Beef Jerky

(Ready in about 4hrs | Servings 10 | Normal)

Ingredients:

- 1-pound of flat iron beef, thinly sliced

- 1/4 cup of soy sauce

- 2 teaspoons of Worcestershire sauce

- 1/4 teaspoon of crushed red pepper flakes

- 1/4 teaspoon of garlic powder

- 1/4 teaspoon of onion powder

Directions:

1. Put all ingredients in a plastic bag or sealed jar and marinate in the refrigerator for 2 hours.

2. Put each jerky slice in a single layer onto the AirFryer shelf.
3. Set the temperature to 160° F and change the timer for 4 hours.
4. Store up to 1 week in airtight containers.

Nutrition: Calories: 85, Protein: 10.2 g, Fiber: 0.0 g, Net Carbohydrates: 0.6 g Fat: 3.5 g, Sodium: 387 mg, Carbohydrates: 0.6 g sugar: 0.2 g.

13. Pork Rind Nachos

(Ready in about 10 min | Servings 2 | Easy)

Ingredients:

- 1-ounce of pork rinds

- 4 ounces of shredded cooked chicken

- 1/2 cup of shredded Monterey jack cheese

- 1/4 cup of sliced pickled jalapeños

- 1/4 cup of guacamole

- 1/4 cup of full-Fat: sour cream

Directions:

1. Put pork rinds in a 6 "round baking pan. Fill with grilled chicken and Monterey cheese jack. Place the pan in the basket with the AirFryer.

2. Set the temperature to 370° F and set the timer for 5 minutes or until the cheese has been melted.
3. Eat right away with jalapeños, guacamole, and sour cream.
4. Enjoy!

Nutrition: Calories: 395, Protein: 30.1 g, Fiber: 1.2 g, Net Carbohydrates: 1.8 g Fat: 27.5 g, Sodium: 763 mg, Carbohydrates: 3.0 g sugar: 1.0 g.

14. Ranch Roasted Almonds

(Ready in about 10 min | Servings 1 | Easy)

Ingredients:

- 2 cups of raw almonds

- 2 tablespoons of unsalted butter, melted

- 1/2 (1-ounce) ranch dressing mix packet

Directions:

1. Swirl the almonds in a wide bowl in butter to cover uniformly. Sprinkle ranch blend and sprinkle over almonds — place almonds in the basket for AirFryer.
2. Set the temperature to 320° F and change the timer for 6 minutes.

3. Shake a basket during the preparation, two to three times.
4. Let it cool off for at least 20 minutes. During refrigeration, almonds may be smooth to become crunchier. Place up to 3 days in an air-tightened jar.
5. Enjoy!

Nutrition: Calories: 190, Protein: 6.0 g, Fiber: 3.0 g, Net Carbohydrates: 4.0 g Fat: 16.7 g, Sodium: 133 mg, Carbohydrates: 7.0 g sugar: 1.0 g.

15. Loaded Roasted Broccoli

(Ready in about 20 min | Servings 2 | Easy)

Ingredients:

- 3 cups of fresh broccoli florets

- 1 tablespoon of coconut oil

- 1/2 cup of shredded sharp Cheddar cheese

- 1/4 cup of full-Fat: sour cream

- 4 slices of sugar-free bacon, cooked and crumbled

- 1 scallion, sliced

Directions:

1. Bring the broccoli into the AirFryer tank and drizzle it with coconut oil.

2. Set the temperature to 350° F and change the timer 10 minutes longer.
3. Toss a basket for two or three times during the training or avoid burning spots.
4. Remove from the fryer as the broccoli continues to crisp at the top. Cover to garnish with melted cheese, sour cream, and crumbled slices of bacon and scallion.

Nutrition: Calories: 361, Protein: 18.4 g, Fiber: 3.6 g, Net Carbohydrates: 6.9 g Fat: 25.7 g, Sodium: 564 mg, Carbohydrates: 10.5 g, Sugar: 3.3 g.

Chapter 3.
Vegetable and
Vegetarian Recipes

16. Cheese and Bean

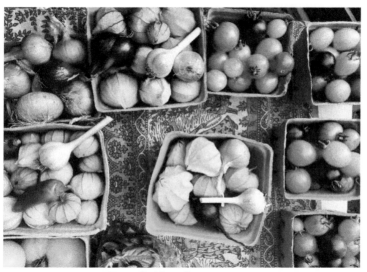

Enchiladas

(Ready in about 35 min | Servings 2
| Normal)

Ingredients:

- Flour tortillas (as many as required)

Red sauce:

- 4 tbsp. of olive oil

- 1 ½ tsp. of garlic that has been chopped

- 1 ½ cups of readymade tomato puree

- 3 medium tomatoes. Puree them in a mixer

- 1 tsp. of sugar

- A pinch of salt or to the taste

- A few red chili flakes to sprinkle

- 1 tsp. of oregano

Filling:

- 2 tbsp. of oil

- 2 tsp. of chopped garlic

- 2 onions chopped finely

- 2 capsicums chopped finely

- 2 cups of readymade baked beans

- A few drops of Tabasco sauce

- 1 cup of crumbled or roughly mashed cottage cheese (cottage cheese)

- 1 cup of grated cheddar cheese

- A pinch of salt

- 1 tsp. of oregano

- ½ tsp. of pepper

- 1 ½ tsp. of red chili flakes or to taste

- 1 tbsp. of finely chopped jalapenos

To serve:

- 1 cup of grated pizza cheese (mix mozzarella and cheddar cheese)

Directions:

1. Prepare tortillas to cook.
2. Now move on to red sauce making. Place about 2 tbsp into a saucepan: heat and stir in the garlic. Attach the remaining ingredients under the heading "For the sauce" Keep going. Cook before sauce drops get dense.
3. Heat one tbsp of oil for filling in another saucepan. Attach onions and garlic, then fry until caramelized or golden-brown color. Connect the remaining ingredients to the filling and cook for two minutes
4. Take the saucepan from the blaze and grate some cheese over the pan. Mix well, and encourage it to settle for a bit.
5. Let's have the platter set. Take a tortilla, then add some

of the surface sauce. Now put the filling in a line at the bottom. Carefully turn the tortilla upwards. And the same for tortillas all around.

6. Now put all the tortillas in a tray and sprinkle with the grated cheese on them. Cover with an aluminum sheet over this.

7. Preheat up the AirFryer for 4-5 minutes at 160° C. Break the bowl and inside the tray. Hold the fryer on for another 15 minutes at the same time. To have a standard cook turn the tortillas over in between.

Nutrition: Calories: 35.

17. Veg Momos

(Ready in about 30 min | Servings 2 | Normal)

Ingredients:

For dough:

- 1 ½ cup of all-purpose flour

- ½ tsp. of salt or to taste

- 5 tbsp. of water

For filling:

- 2 cup of carrots grated

- 2 cup of cabbage grated

- 2 tbsp. of oil

- 2 tsp. of ginger-garlic paste

- 2 tsp. of soy sauce

- 2 tsp. of vinegar

Directions:

1. Knead and cover the dough with plastic wrap, then set aside. Then, prepare the filling ingredients, and strive to make sure the vegetables are well coated with the sauce.
2. Print out the dough, then cut it into a rectangle. Place the center filling. Fold the dough now to protect the filling, then pinch the corners.
3. Preheat up the AirFryer 5 minutes at 200° F. Place the gnocchi's in and close the fry box. Let them cook for another 20 minutes, at the same time. Recommended sides contain chili or ketchup sauce.

Nutrition: Calories: 230 kcal.

18. Cornflakes French Toast

(Ready in about 20 min | Servings 2 | Normal)

Ingredients:

- Bread slices (brown or white)

- 1 egg white for every 2 slices

- 1 tsp. of sugar for every 2 slices

- Crushed cornflakes

Directions:

1. Put together two slices, then cut them around the diagonal. Whisk the egg whites in a mug, then add a little honey.
2. In this mixture, dip the bread triangles and cover with the crushed corn blossoms.
3. Preheat AirFryer for 4 minutes at 180° C. Place the coated bread triangles in and close the fry box. Let them cook temperature likewise for at least another 20 minutes.
4. Switch the triangles over to get an even cook. Serve

chocolate sauce on these
slices.

Nutrition: Calories: 215 kcal.

19. Mint Galette

(Ready in about 10 min | Servings 2
| Easy)

Ingredients:

- 2 cups of mint leaves (Sliced
  fine)

- 2 medium potatoes boiled
  and mashed

- 1 ½ cup of coarsely crushed
  peanuts

- 3 tsp. of ginger finely
  chopped

- 1-2 tbsp. of fresh coriander
  leaves

- 2 or 3 green chilies finely
  chopped

- 1 ½ tbsp. of lemon juice

- Salt and pepper to the taste

Directions:

1. Mix in a clean bowl the sliced mint leaves with the remaining ingredients. Form this mixture into flat and round galettes.
2. Wet the galettes with water gently. Cover with smashed galette each peanut.
3. Preheat the AirFryer for 5 minutes, at 160° Fahrenheit. Place the galettes in the frying bowl and let them steam for another 25 minutes at just the same temperature.
4. Keep turning them around to get a cook that is even. Serve with chutney, basil, or ketchup.

Nutrition: Calories: 150 kcal.

20. Cottage Cheese Sticks

(Ready in about 10 min | Servings 2 | Easy)

Ingredients:

- 2 cups of cottage cheese

- 1 big lemon-juiced

- 1 tbsp. of ginger-garlic paste

- For seasoning, use salt and red chili powder in small amounts

- ½ tsp. of carom

- One or two papadums

- 4 or 5 tbsp. of cornflour

- 1 cup of water

Directions:

1. Take the cheese and cut it into long fragments.

Currently, to use as a marinade, render a mixture of lemon juice, red chili powder, spices, ginger garlic paste, and carom.

2. Let the slices of cottage cheese marinate in the mixture for a while and then roll them in dry cornflour, around 20 minutes, to set them behind.

3. Take the papadum into a saucepan and roast. Crush them into very small bits until they are fried. Now take another bottle and dump about 100 ml of water into it.

4. Loosen 2 tbsp of cornflour in this water. In this cornflour solution, dip the cottage cheese bits and roll them onto the bits of crushed papadum so that the papadum binds to the cottage cheese.

5. About 290 Fahrenheit, preheat the AirFryer for 10 minutes. Then open the fryer basket and put the bits of

cottage cheese inside it. Close well the bowl. Let the fryer sit for another 20 minutes, at 160°.

6. Halfway through, open the basket and throw around a little of the cottage cheese to allow for standard cooking. You should eat it with either ketchup or mint chutney until they're cooked. Serve with mint chutney.

Nutrition: Calories: 175 kcal.

21. Palak Galette

(Ready in about 20 min | Servings 2 | Easy)

Ingredients:

- 2 tbsp. of garam masala

- 2 cups of palak leaves

- 1 ½ cup of coarsely crushed peanuts

- 3 tsp. of ginger finely chopped

- 1-2 tbsp. of fresh coriander leaves

- 2 or 3 green chilies finely chopped

- 1 ½ tbsp. of lemon juice

- Salt and pepper to the taste

Directions:

1. Blend the ingredients into a sterile tub. Form this mixture into flat and circular galettes. Wet the galettes with water gently. Coat with crushed peanuts on each galette.
2. Preheat the AirFryer for 5 minutes, at 160° Fahrenheit. Place the galettes in the fry basket and allow them to cook at the same temperature for another 25 minutes. Go turning them over to get to fry. Serve with ketchup or mint chutney.

Nutrition: Calories: 178 kcal.

22. Spinach Pie

(Ready in about 10 min | Servings 2 | Easy)

Ingredients:

- 7 ounces of flour
- 2 tablespoons of butter
- 7 ounces of spinach
- 1 tablespoon of olive oil
- 2 eggs
- 2 tablespoons of milk
- 3 ounces of cottage cheese
- Salt and black pepper to the taste
- 1 yellow onion, chopped

Directions:

1. Mix the flour and butter, 1 egg, milk, salt, and pepper in your food processor, blend

properly, move to a cup, knead, cover, and leave for 10 minutes.
2. Heat a pan over medium heat with the oil, add the onion and spinach, stir and cook for 2 minutes.
3. Add salt, pepper, leftover egg, and cottage cheese, stir well, and heat up.
4. Divide the dough into 4 bits, roll each slice, place it on the bottom of a ramekin, apply the spinach filling over the dough, put the ramekins in the basket of your AirFryer, and cook for 15 minutes at 360° F.
5. Serve warm.

Enjoy!
Nutrition: Calories: 250, Fat: 12g, Fiber: 2g, Carbs: 23g, Protein: 12g.

23. Balsamic Artichokes

(Ready in about 10 min | Servings 7 | Easy)

Ingredients:

- 4 big artichokes, trimmed

- Salt and black pepper to the taste

- 2 tablespoons of lemon juice

- ¼ cup of extra virgin olive oil

- 2 teaspoons of balsamic vinegar

- 1 teaspoon of oregano, dried

- 2 garlic cloves, minced

Directions:

1. Season the artichokes with salt and pepper, rub them with half the oil and half the lemon juice, place them in

your AirFryer and cook for 7 minutes at 360° F.

2. In the meantime, mix the remaining lemon juice with vinegar, the remaining oil, salt, pepper, garlic, and oregano in a bowl and stir very well.

3. Arrange artichokes on a plate, cut the balsamic vinaigrette over them, and eat.

4. Enjoy!

Nutrition: Calories: 200, Fat: 3g, Fiber: 6g, Carbs: 12g, Protein: 4g.

Chapter 4. Pork, Beef, and Lamb Recipes

24. Pork Chops and

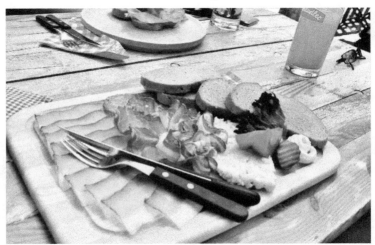

Sage Sauce

(Ready in about 25 min | Servings 2 | Normal)

Ingredients:

- Two Pork cuts

- Salt and black chili, to satisfy

- One tbs of olive oil

- Two tbs of butter

- One Thin shallot

- One Pocket sage, shredded

- One Lemon juice in a teaspoon

Directions:

1. Season pork chops with salt and pepper, season with oil, and place in the AirFryer and continue to for ten minutes at 370 °F, slicing them in the quarter.
2. Besides that, prepare a saucepan on moderate flame with butter, incorporate shallot, two minutes to stir and prepare.
3. Attach sage and lemon juice, mix well, simmer for a couple more minutes before taking some heat off.

4. Start dividing lamb ribs into bowls, drizzle herb sauce, and place all across.
5. Enjoy!

Nutrition: Calories: 265, Fat: 6g, fruit 8, Carbohydrates 19g, Protein: 12g

25. Green Beans and Pork Ribs

(Ready in about 25 min | Servings 4 | Normal)

Ingredients:

- Four chops of pork

- Two lbs. of olive oil

- One tbs of sage, minced

- Salt and black chili, to satisfy

- Sixteen ounces of green beans

- Three cloves of garlic, minced

- Two tbs of parsley, minced

Directions:

1. Mix pork ribs with olive oil, basil, lime in a saucepan which suits your AirFryer, put pepper, green beans,

parsley, and garlic, shake, place in the AirFryer and fry for fifteen min, at 360° F.
2. On plates, split all, and eat.
3. Enjoy!

Nutrition: Calories: 261, Fat: 7g, Carbohydrates 9g, sugars 14g, Protein: 20g.

26. Roasted Pork Chops and Peppers

(Ready in about 26 min | Servings 4 | Normal)

Ingredients:

- Three lbs of olive oil

- Three spoons of lemon juice

- One spoonful of smoked paprika

- Two teaspoons of thyme, minced

- Three cloves of garlic, minced

- Four chops of pork, bone-in

- Salta and black chili, to try

- Two roasted sliced bell peppers

Directions:

1. Mix pork ribs with grease, lemon juice in a saucepan that suits your AirFryer
2. Stir in your AirFryer, the smoked paprika, thyme, garlic, chilies, salt, and pepper, stir well and fry for sixteen minutes at 400° F.
3. Mix pork chops and peppers on bowls, then serve promptly.
4. Enjoy!

Nutrition: Calories: 321, Fat: 6g, Fiber: 8g, Carbohydrates 14g, Protein: 17g.

27. Balsamic Beef

(Ready in about 1hr 10 min | Servings 6 | Difficult)

Ingredients:

- One medium roast beef

- One spoonful of Worcestershire sauce

- 1/2 cup of balsamic vinegar

- One cup stock of beef

- One spoonful of honey

- One pound of soy sauce

- Four cloves of garlic, diced

Directions:

1. Comb roast and bake in a heatproof dish that suits your AirFryer.
2. Add Worcestershire sauce, vinegar, reserve, sugar, garlic, and soy sauce, toss

well in your AirFryer, and bake for 1 hour at 370° F.

3. Break the roast, move between the bowls, scatter the sauce all over and eat.

4. Enjoy!

Nutrition: Calories: 311, Fat: 7g, fruit 12, Carbohydrates 20g, Protein: 16g.

28. Beef Medallions Blend

(Ready in about 2 hr 10 min | Servings 4 | Difficult)

Ingredients:

- Two tablespoons of chili powder

- One basket of tomatoes, smashed

- Four beef medallions

- 2 tsp of onion powder

- 2 tsp of soy sauce

- Salt and black chili, to satisfy

- One tsp of hot pepper

- Two spoonfuls of lime juice

Directions:

1. Blend the tomatoes in a bowl with the hot pepper, soy

sauce, chili powder, onion powder, a tablespoon of salt, lime juice, and black pepper. Whisk fine.

2. Adjust beef medallions in a bowl, sprinkle sauce over them, stir and put them on for 2 hours.
3. Dispose of tomato marinade, place the beef in the AirFryer and cook for ten min, at 360° Fahrenheit
4. On bowls, split steaks and serve with a side salad.
5. Enjoy!

Nutrition: Calories: 230, Fat: 4g, Fiber: 1g, Carbohydrates 13g, Protein: 14g.

29. Mediterranean Scallops and Steaks

(Ready in about 24 min | Servings 2 | Normal)

Ingredients:

- Ten scallops in sea

- Two rainbow steaks

- Four cloves of garlic, minced

- One shallot, cut

- Two tbs. of lemon juice

- Two peregrinated spoons, chopped

- Two tbs. of basil, minced

- One tsp. of lemon zest

- One cup and a half of butter

- 1/4 cup of vegetable reserve

- Salt and black chili, to the taste

Directions:

1. Brush the steaks with salt and pepper, drop them in the fryer and bake for ten min, at 360 °F and switch to a bowl that suits the Fryer.
2. Apply shallot, garlic, butter, basil, lemon juice, parsley. Toss all with zest and scallops, and cook at 360 °F for about four minutes.
3. Split steaks between plates and start serving with scallops.
4. Enjoy!

Nutrition: Calories: 150, Fat: 2g, food 2, Carbohydrates 14g, Protein: 17g.

Chapter 5. Fish and Sea Food

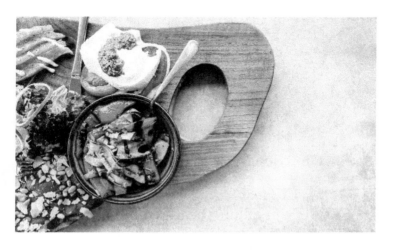

30. Tasty French Cod

(Ready in about 32 min | Servings 4 | Normal)

Ingredients:

- 2 tsp of olive oil

- 1 yellow onion, sliced

- White wine: 1/2 cup

- 2 cloves of garlic, minced

- 14 ounces of dried, stewed tomatoes

- 3 teaspoons of parsley

- 2 lbs. of cod, boneless

- Salt and black chili, to try

- 2 tablespoons of butter

Directions:

1. Heat a saucepan over medium heat with the oil, add garlic and onion, stir, and just cook for five minutes.
2. Insert wine, stir and proceed to cook for 1 minute.
3. Stir in tomatoes, bring to a boil, simmer for 2 minutes, add fuel, stir. Then turn the sun off again.
4. Form of this combination into a heat-proof dish that suits your fryer, add chicken, season with salt and pepper

and steam 350° F in your
fryer for fourteen minutes.
5. Divide the tomatoes and the
fish into plates and serve.
6. Enjoy!

Nutrition: Calories: 231, Fat: 8g,
Fiber: 12g, Carbohydrates 26g,
Protein: 14g.

31. Oriental Fish

(Ready in about 22 min | Servings 4 | Normal)

Ingredients:

- 2 lbs of red snapper fillets, knobbles

- Salt and black chili, to try

- Three cloves of garlic, minced

- One yellow onion, sliced

- One tamarind paste cubic

- 1 tablespoon of oriental sesame oil

- 1 tsp of ginger, grated

- 2 cups of water

- 1/2 cumin cubicle, land

- 1 tsp of lemon juice

- 3 mint spoons, chopped

Directions:

1. Mix the garlic with the onion, salt, pepper, and tamarind in your mixing bowl. Add the paste, sesame oil, ginger, cumin, and water, pulse well, and scrub the fish with that combination.
2. Place the fish at 320° F in your preheated AirFryer and cook for 12 minutes halfway, tossing fish.
3. Divide fish over bowls, chop lemon juice, sprinkle mint, and serve immediately.
4. Enjoy!

Nutrition: Calories: 241, Fat: 8g, Fiber: 16g, Carbohydrates 17g, Protein: 12g.

32. Salmon with Blackberry Glaze

(Ready in about 43 min | Servings 4 | Normal)

Ingredients:

- 1 cup of water

- 1 inch of slice of ginger, grated

- 1/2 lemon juice

- 12 ounces of blackberries

- 1 Tsp of olive oil

- One-half cup of sugar

- 4 medium fillets trout, skinless

- Salt and black chili, to try

Directions:

1. Heat up a casserole with water over a moderate flame.

Add ginger, lemon. Stir in the juice and blackberries, bring to a simmer, simmer for 4-5 minutes, extract in a cup, cover, rinse, return to the pan and mix with the sugar.
2. Bring this mixture to a boil over medium-low heat and simmer for 20 minutes.
3. Leave blackberry sauce to cool, sprinkle with salmon, season with salt and pepper, drizzle all over the olive oil and scrape well.
4. Place the fish at 350° F in your preheated AirFryer and cook for 10 minutes; the fish fillets rotated once.
5. Divide into bowls, add each of the leftover blackberry sauce up and serve.
6. Enjoy!

Nutrition: Calories: 312, Fat: 4g, Fiber: 9g, Carbohydrates 19g, Protein: 14g.

33. Swiss Chard and Lemon Sole

(Ready in about 24 min | Servings 4 | Normal)

Ingredients:

- 1 tsp of lemon zest

- Four slices of white bread, quartered,

- 1/4 cup of walnuts, chopped

- Parmesan: 1/4 cup, rubbed

- 4 lbs. of olive oil

- 4 single, boneless fillets

- Salt and black chili, to try

- 4 cups of butter

- 1/4 cup of lemon juice

- 3 spoons of capers

- 2 cloves of garlic, minced

- 2 swiss chard bunches, diced

Directions:

1. Mix the bread with the walnuts, cheese, and lemon zest in your food processor and then pulse well.
2. Apply half of the olive oil, pulse again really good, and set for now aside.
3. Warm the butter over a moderate flame on a saucepan, add lemon juice, salt. Stir well, pepper and capers, add the tuna, and toss.
4. Switch the fish to the basket of your hot oven AirFryer, cover with bread mix, and cook for 14 minutes at 350° F.
5. In the meantime, fire up another saucepan with the remaining oil, add garlic, Swiss chard, salt and pepper, stir gently and simmer for 2 minutes, then turn off.

6. Divide the tuna into plates and serve horizontally with a sautéed chard.
7. Enjoy it!

Nutrition: Calories: 321, Fat: 7, Fiber: 18g, Carbohydrates 27g, Protein: 12g.

34. Branzino Air Fried

(Ready in about 20 min | Servings 4 | Normal)

Ingredients:

- 1 lemon zest, grated

- One orange zest, grated

- 1/2 lemon juice

- 1/2 orange juice

- Salt and black pepper, to satisfy

- 4 medium fillets of branzino, boneless

- 1/2 cup of parsley

- 2 Pounds of olive oil

- A slice of red, ground pepper flakes

Directions:

1. Mix the fish fillets in a large bowl with the citrus zest, orange zest, lemon juice, orange juice, salt, pepper, flakes of oil and pepper, swirl well, pass the filets thoroughly to 350° F on your preheated AirFryer and bake for 10 minutes, one fillet tossing once.
2. Splash fish on bowls, scatter with parsley and serve promptly.
3. Enjoy!

Nutrition: Calories: 261, Fat: 8g, Fiber: 12g, Carbohydrates 21g, Protein: 12g.

Chapter 6. Poultry Recipes

35. Duck Breast and

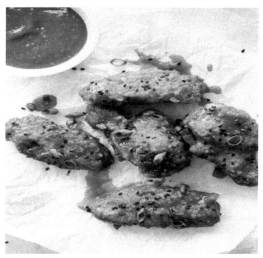

Mango Sauce

(Ready in about 2hr 40 min | Servings 4 | Normal)

Ingredients:

- Four duck breasts

- One and 1/2 lemongrass spoons, sliced

- Three spoons of lemon juice

- Two tsp of olive oil

- Salt and black chili, to satisfy

- Three cloves of garlic, diced

For mango sauce:

- One mango, diced and peeled

- 1 tsp of coriander, chopped

- One red onion, sliced

- One lb of soft chili sauce

- 1 and 1/2 cubic lemon juice

- 1 ginger-spoon, rubbed

- 3/4 cup of sugar

Directions:

1. Comb the duck breasts in a dish of salt, pepper, lemongrass. Toss well with lemon juice, olive oil, and garlic, keep in the refrigerator for 1 hour. Switch to the AirFryer and cook for 10 minutes at 360 °F, one tossing.
2. In the meantime, blend mango with cilantro, onion, chili sauce in a cup, lemon juice, sugar, and ginger, then mix well.
3. Divide the duck into bowls, put a combination of mango on the side, and eat.
4. Enjoy!

Nutrition: Calories: 465, Fat: 11g, fruit 4g, Carbohydrates 29g, Protein: 38g.

36. Chicken Bran and Chili BBQ Sauce

(Ready in about 30 min | Servings 6 | Normal)

Ingredients:

- 2 cups of sauce with chili
- 2 ketchup cups
- 1 cup of jelly pear
- 1/2 teaspoon of smoke solvent
- 1 tablespoon of chili powder
- 1 teaspoon of dried mustard
- 1 teaspoon of tender paprika
- Salt and black chili, to try
- 1 teaspoon of crushed garlic
- Six skinless and boneless chicken breasts

Directions:

1. Season breasts of chicken with salt and pepper, placed in a hot oven AirFryer and cook for ten min, at 350° Fahrenheit.
2. In the meantime, fire up a skillet over medium heat with the chili sauce, add ketchup, pear jelly, butter, smoke with oil, chili powder, mustard powder, paprika, salt, chili pepper and garlic powder. Whisk, then pump it up for 10 minutes.
3. Add the fried chicken breasts to the AirFryer, mix well, split and serve between plates.
4. Enjoy!

Nutrition: Calories: 473, Fat: 13g, fruit 7, Carbohydrates 39g, Protein: 33g.

37. Chicken Breasts Sauce and Passion Fruit

(Ready in about 20 min | Servings 4 | Normal)

Ingredients:

- 4 breasts of chicken

- Salt and black chili, to try

- Four passion fruits, halved, and intended for pulp

- 1 tsp of whisky

- Two tablespoon of star anise

- 2 ounces of maple syrup

- 1 bunch of chives, sliced

Directions:

1. Heat up a saucepan over medium high heat with the passion fruit pulp, incorporate whiskey, star

anise, chives and maple syrup, mix well, cook for 5-6 minutes, and let it off.

2. Rub the chicken with salt and pepper, place the fryer in hot oven air and cook for ten minutes at 360 °F, turning halfway.

3. Split the chicken into bowls, heat the sauce up a little, scatter over the chicken, and then serve.

4. Enjoy!

Nutrition: Calories: 374, Fat: 8g, fruit 22, Carbs: 34g, Protein: 37g.

38. Marinated Ducks Breasts

(Ready in about 1day 15 min | Servings 2 | Normal)

Ingredients:

- Two duck breasts

- One cup of white wine

- 1/4 cup of soy sauce

- Two cloves of garlic, minced

- Six tarragon springs

- Salt and black chili, to satisfy

- 1 pound of butter

- 1/4 classic sherry

Directions:

1. Comb the duck breasts in a dish of white wine, soya sauce, ginger, tarragon, toss well with salt and pepper,

and remain in the refrigerator for 1 day.
2. Switch the duck breasts 350° F to your hot oven AirFryer and cook ten minutes, halfway spinning.
3. In the meantime, pour the marinade into a saucepan, set over medium pressure, add butter and sherry, bring to a boil, simmer for 5 minutes and take off the heat.
4. Divide the duck breasts into bowls, drizzle all over the sauce and eat.
5. Enjoy!

Nutrition: Calories: 475, Fat: 12g, Fiber: 3g, Carbohydrates 10g, Protein: 48g.

39. Duck and Sauce with Tea

(Ready in about 30 min | Servings 4 | Normal)

Ingredients:

- Two and half of breast duck, boneless

- Two and 1/4 cup stocks of chicken

- Shallot: 3/4 cup, chopped

- One and a half cup of orange juice

- Salt and black chili, to try

- Three teaspoons of Earl Gray tea

- Three tsp of butter, melted

- One tablespoon of honey

Directions:

1. Season with salt and pepper in duck breast part, put in hot oven AirFryer. Cook for ten minutes, at 360° Fahrenheit.
2. In the meantime, prepare a saucepan over a moderate flame with butter, add shallot. Remove and boil for 2-3 minutes.
3. Stir in stock and cook for another minute.
4. Include orange juice, tea leaves, and sugar, stir and boil for 2-3 minutes, and put pressure on a tub.
5. Divide the duck into bowls, drizzle all over the tea sauce and eat.
6. Enjoy!

Nutrition: Calories: 228, Fat: 11g, Fiber: 2g, Carbohydrates 20g, Protein: 12g.

40. Simple Duck Breasts

(Ready in about 25 min | Servings 4 | Normal)

Ingredients:

- Four skinless duck breasts

- Four garlic heads, sliced, cut, and diced tops

- 1 cup of lemon juice

- Salt and black chili, to satisfy

- 1/2 cubit of lemon pepper

- 1 1/2 cubic of olive oil

Directions:

1. Mix duck breasts in a garlic dish, lemon juice, salt, chili pepper, and lemon. Add olive oil and pepper, and mix everything.

2. Switch the duck and garlic to the AirFryer and prepare for 15 minutes at 350° F.
3. Divide and scatter duck breasts and garlic on bowls.
4. Enjoy!

Nutrition: Calories: 200, dietary food 7, sugars 11g, Protein: 17g.

Chapter 7. Desserts and Sweets Recipes

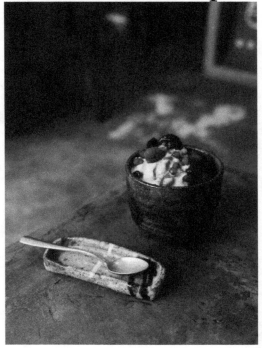

41. Poppyseed Cake

(Ready in about 40 min | Servings 6 | Normal)

Ingredients:

- 1 and a half cups of flour

- 1 teaspoon of powder baking

- 3⁄4 cups of sugar:

- One tablespoon of rubbed orange zest

- Two lime zest, rubbed

- Butter: 1⁄2 cup, mild

- 2 whisked eggs,

- 1⁄2 teaspoon of vanilla extract

- 2 tablespoons of poppy seeds

- 1 cup of milk

To the cream:

- 1 cup of sugar

- 1⁄2 cup of passion fruit puree

- Three tablespoons of butter, melted

- 4 yolks of eggs

Directions:

1. Mix the flour and baking powder in a tub, 3/4 cup sugar, orange zest, and zest lime, then mix.
2. Add 1/2 cup butter, eggs, poppy seeds, vanilla, and milk and blend with your blender load into an air-fried cake pan and cook at 350° F for thirty minutes.
3. In the meantime, fire up a pan over medium heat with three tablespoons of butter. Mix and add sugar till it decomposes.
4. Strip from heat, steadily incorporate the passion fruit puree and egg yolks and whisk well.
5. Remove the cake from the fryer, cool it down a little, and horizontally break into halves.
6. Pour over 1/4 of the passion fruit cream, finish with the other half of the cake and finish with 1/4 of the cream.

7. Serve fresh.
8. Enjoy!

Nutrition: Calories: 211, Fat: 6g, Fiber: 7g, Carbohydrates 12g, Protein: 6g.

42. Pears and Espresso Cream

(Ready in about 40 min | Servings 4 | Normal)

Ingredients:

- 4 half pears, and hulled
- 2 tablespoons of lemon juice
- 1 tablespoon of sugar
- 2 tablespoons of water
- 2 tablespoons of butter

For the creme:

- 1 cup of ice cream
- One cup of mascarpone
- 1/3 cups of sugar
- 2 tablespoons of espresso, cool

Directions:

1. Comb pears half with lemon juice, 1 tablespoon of sugar, and butter in a bowl, including water, stir well, switch to the AirFryer, and cook at 360° F for 30 minutes.
2. In the meantime, blend whipped cream and mascarpone in a tub, 1/3 cup. Whisk sugar and espresso very well and hold in the refrigerator until the pears are prepared.
3. Split pears into bowls, cover with and serve with espresso cream.
4. Enjoy!

Nutrition: Calories: 211, Fat: 5g, Fiber: 7g, Carbohydrates 8g, Protein: 7g.

43. Bars of Lemon

(Ready in about 35 min | Servings 6 | Normal)

Ingredients:

- Four eggs

- 2 and 1/4 cups of flour

- 2 lemon juice

- 1 cup of soft butter

- 2 cups of sugar

Directions:

1. Comb butter in a dish of 1/2 cup of sugar and 2 cups of flour, mix well and push in the fryer and position on the bottom of the pan that suits your AirFryer. Cook for 10 minutes, at 350° F.
2. Comb the rest of the sugar in yet another container with the rest of the flour, the eggs,

and lemon juice, whisk well, scatter all over the crust.

3. Put in the fryer at 350° F for another 15 minutes, set aside the cut bars, cool off, and serve.

4. Enjoy!

Nutrition: Calories: 125, Fat: 4g, carbohydrate 16g, Protein: 2g.

44. Figs and Butter Blend with Coconut

(Ready in about 10 min | Servings 3 | Normal)

Ingredients:

- Two tablespoons of coconut butter

- 12 half-figs

- One and a half cup of sugar

- 1 cup of almonds, fried and chopped

Directions:

1. Put butter in a saucepan that suits your fryer and melt over medium-strong temperature.
2. Include figs, sugar, and almonds, toss, put in your frying pan, and cook 4 minutes at 300° Fahrenheit
3. Serve cool and split into cups.

4. Enjoy!

Nutrition: Calories: 170, Fat: 4g, Fiber: 5g, Carbohydrates 7g, Protein: 9g.

45. Pumpkin Cookies

(Ready in about 25 min | Servings
24 | Normal)

Ingredients:

- Two and a half cups of rice

- 1/2 teaspoon of baking soda

- 1 tablespoon of flaxseed

- 3 tablespoon of water

- 1/2 cup of pumpkin squash,
  mashed

- 1/4 cups of honey

- 2 cups of butter

- 1 teaspoon of vanilla extract

- 1/2 cup of dark chocolate
  chips

Directions:

1. Comb flax seed with water in a tub, swirl, and set aside for a couple of minutes.
2. Mix the flour with the salt and baking soda in another dish.
3. Match the honey and the pumpkin puree, butter, and spice in a separate dish extract and field flax.
4. Combine the flour and the chocolate chips with the honey mixture and whisk.
5. Scoop 1 pound of cookie dough on a rimmed baking sheet. Put in your AirFryer, repeat for the rest of the dough, bring them in the AirFryer, and cook for fifteen minutes at 350° Fahrenheit.
6. Cookies should be left to cool off and serve.
7. Enjoy!

Nutrition: Calories: 140, Fat: 2g, Carbohydrates 7g, Protein: 10g.

46. Air Fried Apples

(Ready in about 37 min | Servings 4 | Normal)

Ingredients:

- Four big, cored apples

- Just a couple of raisins

- 1 tablespoon of cinnamon, ground

- Honey to satisfy

Directions:

1. Fill the apple with raisins, sprinkle cinnamon, chop honey, place in and cook them in the AirFryer and simmer for 17 minutes at 367° F.
2. Let them cool off and then serve.
3. Enjoy!

Nutrition: Calories: 220, Fat: 3g, Fiber: 3g, Carbohydrates 6g, Protein: 10g.

47. Fruit Pudding with Passion

(Ready in about 50 min | Servings 6 | Normal)

Ingredients:

- 1 cup of passion fruit curd

- 4 passion fruits pulp and seeds

- 3 and one-half ounces of maple syrup

- 3 eggs

- 2 ghee ounces, melted

- 3 and one-half ounces of almond milk

- half cup of almond flour

- 1/2 teaspoon of baking powder

Directions:

1. Blend half the fruit curd in a dish with the passion fruit seeds and mix, pulp, and split into Six heat-proof ramekins.
2. Whisked eggs in a tub, with maple syrup, ghee, the rest of the mix excellently: curd, baking powder, milk, and flour.
3. Also, split this into the ramekins, put in the fryer, and cook for 40 minutes at 200° Fahrenheit.
4. Leave the puddings and prepare to cool down!
5. Enjoy!

Nutrition: Calories: 430, Fat: 22g, Fiber: 3g, Carbohydrates g7, Protein: 8g.

48. Mixed Berries

(Ready in about 11 min | Servings 6 | Normal)

Ingredients:

- 2 tablespoons of lemon juice

- 1 and 1⁄2 tablespoons of maple syrup

- 1 and 1⁄2 spoonful of champagne vinegar

- 1 tablespoon of olive oil

- 1 lb. of strawberries, half cut

- 1 and 1⁄2 cups of blueberries

- 1⁄4 cup of basil leaves

Directions:

1. Comb lemon juice with maple syrup in a saucepan which suits your AirFryer. Stir in vinegar, bring to a simmer over a moderate

flame, and add oil. Stir, put the blueberries and strawberries in your AirFryer, and cook 6 minutes, at 310° F.

2. Sprinkle over the basil and serve!
3. Enjoy!

Nutrition: Calories: 163, Fat: 4g, Carbohydrates 4g, Carbohydrates 10g, Protein: 2.1g.

Chapter 8. Lunch Recipes

49. AirFryer Fried Rice

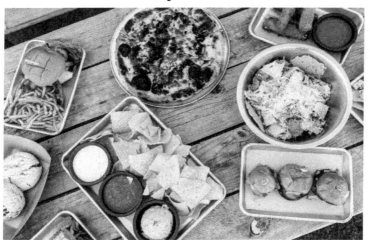

with Sesame-Sriracha Sauce

(Ready in about 40 min | Servings 2 | Normal)

Ingredients

- 2 cups of cooked white rice

- 1 tablespoon of vegetable oil

- 2 teaspoons of toasted sesame oil

- Kosher salt and freshly ground black pepper

- 1 teaspoon of sriracha

- 1 teaspoon of soy sauce

- 1/2 teaspoon of sesame seeds, preferably toasted, plus more for topping

- 1 large egg, lightly beaten

- 1 cup of frozen peas and carrots, thawed

Directions:

1. In a cup, add the rice, vegetable oil, 1 teaspoon sesame oil, and 1 tablespoon water. To brush the rice, season with salt and pepper and throw. Switch to an insert with a 7-inch diameter

AirFryer, metal cake tray, or foil plate.

2. Place the pan in a 5.3-quarter AirFryer and cook for around 12 minutes at 350° F, stirring about halfway until the rice is slightly toasted and crunchy.

3. Meanwhile, in a small bowl, combine the sriracha, soy sauce, sesame seeds, and remaining 1 teaspoon of sesame oil.

4. Open the fryer to the air and dump the rice over the potato. Close and cook for about 4 minutes before the egg is cooked completely. Add the peas and carrots to open again and mix in the rice to spread and break up the potato. Close and cook the peas and carrots for more minutes to heat up.

5. In pans, spoon the fried rice, chop with some of the sauce and scatter with more sesame seeds.

Nutrition: Calories: 475 kcal.

50. Colored Veggie Rice

(Ready in about 35 min | Servings 4 | Normal)

Ingredients:

- 2 cups of basmati rice
- 1 cup of mixed carrots, peas, corn, and green beans
- 2 cups of water
- ½ teaspoon of green chili, minced
- ½ teaspoon of ginger, grated
- 3 garlic cloves, minced
- 2 tablespoons of butter
- 1 teaspoon of cinnamon powder
- 1 tablespoon of cumin seeds
- 2 bay leaves

- 3 whole cloves

- 5 black peppercorns

- 2 whole cardamoms

- 1 tablespoon of sugar

- Salt to the taste

Directions:

1. Put the water in a heat-proof dish that suits your AirFryer; add rice, mixed vegetables, green chili, rubbed ginger, garlic cloves, cinnamon, cloves, butter, cumin seeds, bay leaves, cardamom, black peppercorns, salt, and sugar. Swirl, place in the basket of your AirFryer, and cook for 25 minutes at 370° F.
2. Break into bowls and serve.
3. Enjoy!

Nutrition: Calories: 283, Fat: 4g, Fiber: 8g, Carbs: 34g, Protein: 14g.

Conclusion

In short, from what we can see in all the recipes in this book, we can conclude that frying food in a hot air fryer is a much healthier way of consuming it, compared to traditional oil fryers.

In addition to being much healthier because we avoid eating excess fat, hot air fryers can prepare many meals, they do not limit us at all. Within these fryers that work without oil, we can prepare, in addition to all the products that we would do in a conventional fryer, many more.

Some of these dishes can be as delicious and easy as lemon bars, pizza, and colored veggie rice or delicious (and not at all greasy) chicken wings with french fries. Great and super healthy options!

CPSIA information can be obtained
at www.ICGtesting.com
Printed in the USA
BVHW062032020321
601494BV00010B/826